ROLLERCOASTER RIDE

The aftermath of suicide
Poems for healing, hope
and moving forward

Jo Woodhouse

Rollercoaster Ride
The aftermath of suicide
Poems for healing, hope and moving forward

First published in Australia by Jo Woodhouse 2023
www.jowoodhouse.com

A catalogue record for this
book is available from the
National Library of Australia

ISBN: 978-0-6459418-0-7 (pbk)
ISBN: 978-0-6459418-1-4 (ebk)

Any similarity to other persons' stories, poems or comments,
living or dead, is completely unintentional and coincidental.

Typesetting and design by Publicious Book Publishing
Published in collaboration with Publicious Book Publishing
www.publicious.com.au

Cover image: I-ing © (shutterstock)
Proofread by Julie Guthrie (Publicious)

Dedication

I am so grateful to everyone who has helped bring this book to life, and for those who have supported me through the hardest times.

Introduction

It was World Mental Health Day, and the day the man in my life took his own. In just moments, everything changed. Life became very different.

As I navigated through the aftermath, ultimately I had two choices—I could learn to ride the waves very quickly, or I could drown. I chose to ride the waves, even though I fell off from time to time.

I've never written a book before, but it's been very cathartic. Somehow, poetry helped me make sense of all the different emotions I was dealing with and the events that unfolded after his death. Many things I didn't know beforehand but I realised through this process; it seems I didn't really know him at all.

We also worked together. And being retrenched only months later didn't help and certainly caused me to spiral further. I struggled at first. Who wouldn't? These were two life-changing moments that happened back to back and I didn't get a say in either of them. Walking out of interviews in tears was not ideal, and since then, finding the right company for me has certainly been challenging. And if that wasn't enough, at the time all this was happening, Mum was also battling cancer.

You don't necessarily overcome grief, you somehow find a way to live with it, endure it and slowly heal yourself around the pain as you continue living your life. I am also a very emotional person, which probably doesn't help.

This trauma and the subsequent collateral damage has been life changing, but writing has definitely helped in my healing process. And I think many other emotions of my life have come through in this book.

Considering the increase in deaths by way of suicide worldwide, it's important to continue to talk about this topic. We need to educate and keep the conversation going.

The loss you feel when a loved one dies by suicide is unbearable. It's confronting and it's final. Over the years, I've lost several friends and colleagues due to mental illness, and many feelings from the past resurfaced. Statistics on the Lifeline website show that up to 135 people are exposed each time someone takes their own life. These are family, friends and colleagues who may require the need of clinician services or support following the trauma.

Many people have been affected and I'm not speaking for anyone else involved as we all had different relationships. Everyone's experience is unique and I can only react to things as I know them. I've written these poems from my own emotions, experience, research, shared experiences, and putting myself in other people's shoes. While one event initiated these poems, they are a mix of poems that include losing others with mental illness, dealing with further curveballs back to back, and additional events in life as time goes on.

Originally, I was writing for my own healing; however, several friends suggested that my poems need to be heard and I should publish them. So, here we are. Everyone has a personal story to tell, and these are some chapters in mine.

The ones who take this path don't see the aftermath they leave behind. They don't see the pain and suffering others are left to face, or how they'll continue to struggle in their lives for different reasons. They don't see our rollercoaster ride!

If these poems make just one person realise the ripple effect of pain they would leave behind, hopefully they won't do it.

If they can save just one person's life, it's worth it!

Contents

Denial

This really can't be happening
It simply can't be true
It's so very overwhelming
When they tell me it was you

I don't believe what I'm being told
I don't believe you're gone
I don't believe you took your life
I can't think to carry on

My heart, it just keeps hurting
It's breaking into two
I can't bring myself to believe
Why was it you? Why you?

Loss

I miss you
I miss your hugs
I miss your voice
I miss how you made me feel
My life has changed from day to day
Part of me is missing
My heart hurts
I struggle with pain and anxiety I've never had before
This pain is so great, it's hard to put into words
Nobody really understands
I still talk to you, but I get no reply
I keep looking at my phone, but no calls or messages
I have so many questions
I'm so angry
Plans are cancelled, there's nothing to look forward to
Tears constantly flow from my eyes
I don't know how to deal with this
I'm just lost

Guilt

Guilt consumes us
For not being able to help you
Because we're here and you're not
When we smile or laugh
When we try to enjoy ourselves
Because we should have done more
Because we couldn't get you to really hear us
Guilt builds up inside us
It's unbearable
Guilt continues to play on our minds

Angry

I trusted you not to hurt me
You said you never would
You said you really wanted me
You said that we were good

I made it very clear to you
Not to hurt me from the start
You promised me you wouldn't
And you didn't want to part

You said I'm what you needed
And that you really cared
You said that you were happy
With the things we shared

This was our life, not just yours
It affected both our lives
But you took that choice away from me
The day you chose to die

My heart is filled with so much pain
And I am bereft
You have changed my life forever
I'm so angry that you left

I can't breathe

I wake up in the morning
Wishing you were here with me
I reach out but you're nowhere
I can't breathe

I can't accept you left
And struggle to believe
You didn't think I'd miss you
I can't breathe

I miss the time we spent together
And the way you made me feel
I have such weight upon my chest
I can't breathe

I try to go about my day
But grief's controlling me
The small things seem impossible
I can't breathe

I'm hypnotised with sadness
As emotions smother me
Understanding what just happened
I can't breathe

I live so much with heartbreak
With suffering and grief
There's so much to this story
I can't breathe

I'll struggle with trust and moving on
I'll never be quite me
I hope in time, the pain will ease
But right now, I can't breathe

I wish I saved your life

How can I really know you?
When you bottle up inside
You tell me half the story
Of what's really on your mind

I can't help if I don't know
The pain you really feel
We could have worked together
I could have helped you heal

I wish you could have talked about
What you truly felt inside
Your story, not just parts of it
You didn't have to hide

I really wish you let me know
What was truly in your heart
And what you really struggled with
Because I cared right from the start

I didn't know that you were struggling
I didn't know you were in strife
I wished you cried for help that day
I wished I saved your life

This aftermath

You knew that you were hurting
As you'd been down this path before
But you continued chasing after me
You should have closed that door

You can't see how much you've hurt me
In more ways than one
We cannot change what's happened
'Cause now, what's done is done

I'm now the one who's left behind
And the one who lives in pain
You don't realise what you've done to me
There's nothing left to gain

I live with hurt and sorrow
As I find out more each day
You could have moved on any time
I wasn't forcing you to stay

I don't deserve this kind of treatment
I was always good to you
But it seems you needed more than that
And this behaviour isn't new

You said you only wanted me
But it seems now that's not true
I just found out you have someone else
Who would also be missing you

I made sure you always had support
I checked up on you each day
You had someone who believed in you
Now it seems I have to pay

Let's hope I can be stronger
And not follow down your path
To put others in my shoes now
And have to face this aftermath

This ride

It's a long and lonely journey
Down this track that I'm now on
I just don't want to be here
And still don't believe you've gone

I didn't want to take this ride
And wished you called for help that day
This pain is overwhelming
And I'm trying to be brave

There's so much to this story
I wonder how I'll ever heal
I wish you thought of others that day
And the loss that we all feel

It's clear that you were troubled
Needing different people in your life
We could've all come together
And supported you through the strife

Some days are just unbearable
There's so much pain inside
This track seems never-ending
Why did you make me take this ride?

The ripple effect

You tossed the stone across the water
The ripples on their way
The ripples mean there's no way back
And fate was had that day

The ripples wavered outwards
There was no point of return
But you can't see below the water
Or your presence for which we yearn

The stone sinks to the bottom
Taking our hearts with it too
But you don't see the stone has changed us
As we face life without you

The ripples hurt so many people
And they show you were in strife
But this action bears a consequence
'Cause the ripples last for life

You must have thought nobody loved you
Or maybe nobody cared
But you were loved and you were wanted
You must have been so scared

The world turns all around us now
But we keep standing still
Our lives will never be the same
Because of the place you filled

I wish you could see the turmoil
And the void you've left behind
That we never would have left you
And you're always on our mind

We now live with anxiety
And we have ongoing pain
It's so hard moving forward
As our sun has turned to rain

We have unanswered questions
Our blue sky has turned to grey
Our tears come out of nowhere
And we still struggle day to day

We wished you came and talked with us
We would have given you our time
We would have all supported you
And helped your stars align

We didn't get the chance to help you
You didn't even let us try
To help us understand your pain
You left with no goodbye

The pain we have won't leave us now
We'll just carry it day to day
You didn't think it would affect us
But it will never go away

We wish you didn't take this path
And you were still here in our lives
You will always be remembered
Because we'll never say 'goodbye'

But it seems you didn't see the outcome
And as I now reflect
I guess you didn't think about
The lifelong ripple effect

Unfinished business

We had unfinished business
Because you didn't say goodbye
You didn't tell me you were leaving
You didn't even try

We had unfinished business
We had things to discuss
Your decision wasn't just for you
It affected both of us

We had unfinished business
We had hopes and we had plans
You didn't let us finish them
I'll never really understand

We had unfinished business
There were things you should have said
But you kept your actions private
You should have opened up instead

We had unfinished business
But it's no longer about us
Questions always cloud my mind
But they'll never be discussed

Log a ticket please

Our work is like a ghost town
It's eerie and it's quiet
It's nothing like it used to be
It's sad and not quite right

There's such a different feeling now
It's hard to work from there
It's hard to walk past where you sat
And see your empty chair

Our colleagues are all hurting
As they're feeling this pain too
The office is just not the same
It's different without you

I talk to many people
And they share a tale or two
They think about you often
As they're also missing you

If only we could hear your voice
And put our minds at ease
If only we could hear you say
'Log a ticket please'

When you leave

You were a dedicated worker
You had respect and you had trust
You were kind and you were loyal
And you were always there for us

You used to work so many hours
And at night you'd pace the halls
Checking everything's in order
Between late night conference calls

You did the best thing for the company
With so many things achieved
You will always be remembered
Turn the lights off when you leave

Without you

The first night I spent without you
I was in pain and disbelief
I can't comprehend what happened
And now live with so much grief

The next night I spent without you
Was no better than before
As day and night turns into one
I miss you even more

I keep fighting nights without you
As I have no other choice
I wish you were here to hold me tight
I wish I could hear your voice

I'm tired of nights without you
And I really wish you knew
I don't know how to handle this
And fight another night without you

The road we chose

You can't see through the darkness
You can't see past your pain
The turmoil and confusion
But you had so much to gain

We know you had a broken heart
But you were generous and kind
You were filled with much emotion
But darkness clouds your mind

You had love that surrounded you
But we couldn't make you see
That your life was so important
But you seemed to disagree

We wish you didn't take this ending
Or make us take this ride
There's so many people hurting now
It just tears us up inside

Your depression must have changed you
And made you just withdraw
From family, friends and life itself
You couldn't take it anymore

You could no longer fight your battle
And brought your life to a close
But the ones left behind are suffering
And it's not the road we chose

Me

I'm me, but I'm not me
I'm different now, my personality is not the same
I'm broken
I continue to feel sad and empty
I feel nauseous all the time
I've lost so much weight
There's too many curveballs back to back
It's hard to keep up
There's a constant ache in the pit of my stomach
I'm happy in some moments, but I'm not happy
I laugh sometimes, but it's a hollow laugh
I smile at times, but it's not a true smile
I feel like I'm still dying on the inside
I don't know when the real me will return
I don't even know if it will
It will be a different me
I have to find a new meaning of life
I have to learn to breathe, trust, laugh, and live again

I couldn't walk away

I couldn't walk away from you
When you told me of your pain
I said I'd walk beside you
And help you through the strain

You said you needed me to help you
And thanked me for being there
You thanked me for supporting you
And showing that I care

Some days I walked on egg shells
When you thought you weren't worthwhile
But we had some happy moments
When I could make you smile

Some days you had such sadness
Some days you had some tears
In times you tried to open up
And share your biggest fears

Sometimes it wasn't perfect
And there were struggles day to day
But your life was important
And I couldn't walk away

The grief train

The grief train departs the station
As my time with you is gone
It's a ride of mixed emotions
It's not the train I should be on

It rides the track of ups and downs
Of anger, loss and guilt
Of rejection, hurt and emptiness
Where is the life we built?

It heads into the tunnel
Where you feel there's no way out
There's no light at the end of it
There's just many clouds of doubt

It's a journey full of sadness
It's a long and lonely ride
No one really understands it
Or feels this pain I have inside

As we pull into the station
I wish this ride came to a close
I didn't want this ticket
It's not the track I chose

I just want to end this journey
I didn't want it from the start
Please help me get a refund
So you never break my heart

The storm

I wasn't gonna leave you
When you needed me the most
'Cause if you struggled through the day
I needed to stay close

I promised I'd support you
And I'd help you through the storm
But the clouds rolled in and made it tough
The lightning struck a chord

I wish you reached out in the whirlwind
I would've been right by your side
To wait until the storm had passed
I would've helped you through this ride

It must have been a masterpiece
The thunder filled your mind
You couldn't see that calm would come
Or the solace you might find

The eye of the storm was just so dark
The full impact took effect
You couldn't endure the hurricane
It seems you had nothing left

I wish you chose to weather it
And fought with strength and form
But I guess it overwhelmed you
And you couldn't fight the storm

Missing you this Christmas

I'm missing you this Christmas
As I look up at the sky
Tonight I light a candle
And wish you didn't say goodbye

I'm missing you this Christmas
And I dream of better times
When life was not so painful
I have so much on my mind

I'm missing you this Christmas
And I long for days gone by
Wishing you didn't take this path
As I hide my pain inside

I'm missing you this Christmas
And try not to show my tears
To enjoy time with my family
And the ones that I hold dear

I'm missing you this Christmas
Wish I changed what you went through
To really take your pain away
Would be my Christmas gift to you

A new year without you

I look back on the year gone by
As a new year soon will rise
I reflect on what life brought me
And remember happy times

I'll set a plan of goals and dreams
And complete ones we didn't do
Maybe they're not all possible
As they no longer include you

Tomorrow when the dawn will break
And the new year comes to start
I'll think of you as I always do
As you're locked inside my heart

So, as the year comes to an end
And when the night is through
The sun will rise and shine again
As I start a new year without you

We didn't have a choice

You left us without notice
You didn't say goodbye
Part of us went with you
With tears tonight we cry

We weren't ready for this road
We're all left with so much pain
You were loved and you were wanted
But you didn't die in vain

Your mind must have been so dark
You couldn't see the light
But what you didn't realise
Your aura shone so bright

You used to always make us laugh
You used to make us smile
We enjoyed spending our time with you
You had your unique style

We know we couldn't feel your pain
It's something we can't see
We hope you're in a peaceful place
Now that you've been set free

You couldn't keep the battle
And we couldn't hear your voice
You finally gave up fighting
But we didn't have a choice

The sea of grief

I'm drowning in the sea of grief
I can't catch my breath
The waves are crashing over me
But I have nothing left

I scream out for a lifeguard
But nobody hears my call
The waves continue to pull me under
There's no one there at all

I try to keep my head afloat
But life just keeps me down
These curveballs are just all too great
I feel that I will drown

The waves continue to crash on me
Of rejection, loss and pain
I just don't have the energy
To fight these waves again

This rollercoaster ride

How can I make you understand?
This journey that I'm on
The pain, the loss, the sorrow
My life and how it's gone

How can I make you understand?
The grief that I now feel
The days of mixed emotions
And the sadness as I heal

How can I make you understand?
It's a long and lonely ride
Some days are just unbearable
As I deal with pain inside

How can I make you understand?
My interest now has gone
I try hard to stay focused
But it's so hard moving on

How can I make you understand?
I don't know what you say
I try but I can't hear you
I'm just getting through the day

How can I make you understand?
I might look like I am well
The reality is I'm struggling
In my own living hell

How can I make you understand?
I just fake it through the day
My laugh, my smile, my happiness
Have all just gone away

How can I make you understand?
How this grief's affected me
What it's like in my shoes now
And how it's made me be

How can I make you understand?
I show you a difference face
One for show and one for home
I feel so out of place

How can I make you understand?
When there's nothing I can say
To ever make you really know
How I truly feel each day

I can never make you understand
The pain and loss inside
This long and lonely journey
This rollercoaster ride

Each day

Each day is a new journey
As I travel down this path
It's days of mixed emotions
Working through this aftermath

Each day I wake up lonely
And realise that you've gone
I take one big step backwards
As I remember to move on

Each day I take that one deep breath
And go about my day
But I wonder how things might have been
If I could've made you stay

Each day I take it step by step
As I try to look ahead
I have to just look forward
And rebuild my life instead

Each day I don't get answers
To the questions on my mind
I need to deal with letting go
For some closure I must find

Each day I have my checklist
Of all things that I must do
This helps me take steps forward
In a new life without you

Each day I just keep going
And take one step at a time
I thank God for those supporting me
And the good things in my life

I know in time the pain will fade
It's what I must believe
That life goes on, and in my thoughts
You'll be a memory

What will tomorrow bring?

Emptiness surrounds me
As I remember days with you
Now they're only memories
Of the man that I once knew

But I guess I didn't really know
That much about your life
You only showed me part of you
And now it cuts just like a knife

You painted me a different picture
Of what life was all about
About how much I meant to you
But now I have such doubt

You left me without notice
And to deal with so much grief
You left me to pick up pieces
There just seems no relief

It's hard to understand what happened
And what I know now since you died
It seems you told me stories
And now I know you lied

You left me to deal with so much pain
I feel I didn't mean a thing
And day by day I find out more
What will tomorrow bring?

Don't tell me how to grieve

Please don't tell me how to grieve
You're not walking in my shoes
You're not on this journey
I don't need someone else's views

You might think you're coming from a place of heart
But you don't know what it's like
You don't know the story
You don't know the aftermath

You don't realise that I'm dealing with
More than one event in life
My world has been turned upside down
You don't realise I'm in strife

Don't tell me to be happy
When so much of life is gone
You don't know I was retrenched today
It's not so easy to move on

This really isn't helpful
And it just makes me mad
When people think they know my needs
Maybe I need a hand

Don't think you know what's best for me
Or that I should hide my pain
My life is filled with emptiness
My sun has turned to rain

Grief can last a lifetime
It's an isolating ride
There's much more to this story
And I have such pain inside

So, walk with me and be my friend
And help me through this time
I need you to be supportive
With the mountain I must climb

I'll always ride with you

You shared with me your passion
You taught me how to ride
You bought my bike and all the gear
We'd go riding side by side

We'd race each other down the hills
You'd chase me up the other side
I'd feel the wind blow through my hair
And the sunshine while we ride

We booked the ride to Wollongong
You said it's what you loved to do
I had a team who rode with me
But crossed the finish line without you

They will be much-loved memories
When it was just us two
I'll continue with your passion
And I'll always ride with you

If I could paint your picture

If I could paint your picture
It would not be black and white
I would paint it full of colour
I'd paint you a different life

If I could paint your picture
First, I'd paint your eyes
I'd make sure that they sparkled
And they never had to cry

If I could paint your picture
I'd then paint your smile
I would make it shine so brightly
I would make you feel worthwhile

If I could paint your picture
I would paint your caring heart
I'd make sure that nothing broke it
So you'd never fall apart

If I could paint your picture
I would paint you whole again
I would ensure that nothing hurt you
And you never felt such pain

Your puzzled life

Your life was such a puzzle
And we were all one part
It was many different pieces
The full story in your heart

There were many different colours
And many puzzle shapes
This gave you a distraction
This gave you an escape

The puzzle would have changed you
And got more complex through the years
With interlocking pieces
That hid your biggest fears

It must have been so convoluted
But you seemed to have the skill
To try and piece it all together
So you didn't seem so ill

Your puzzle was a mystery
With every passing day
What was the final picture?
What would it look like if you stayed?

Your final day

Your world's no longer dark now
As you move towards the light
Because of the path you went down
You gave up the will to fight

I wonder how you really felt
And what you thought on your last day
Did you feel some satisfaction
That your pain was on its way?

The light was getting closer
The darkness fades away
You probably felt your pain escape
On what was your final day

I will never forget the day you left
It's embedded in my heart
It was the day before my birthday
That you tore my world apart

So, on my birthday every year
It pains me now to say
I'll be constantly reminded
When you left that final day

The sun sets on your life

The dark stops you from sleeping
And you stir throughout the night
Thoughts constantly keeping you awake
As you see the morning light

A new dawn will rise to meet you
And you greet another day
But a new day keeps you fighting
You want the pain to go away

You continue with your turmoil
But keep silent in your pain
You don't share all your feelings
And you struggle with the strain

You go about your business
And just get through the day
But with every passing sunrise
Your sky is always grey

As the sun rose on your final day
You no longer feel in strife
And as you now have freed your mind
The sun sets on your life

Depression is invisible

For those living with depression
It was very hard to hear
The stories that they told me
As some shared their biggest fears

Depression is invisible
You can't see a visual sign
It's a constant daily battle
And it's exhausting all the time

I'm always drained and tired
It's grueling every day
People tell me to 'snap out of it'
It doesn't help in any way

I come across a bubbly person
But I'm sad and I'm alone
No one sees the tears I cry
When I'm on my own

I come across as witty
And I crack jokes constantly
I try to be the funny person
So no one sees the real me

I'm very antisocial
And I don't want to speak
I hide in my phone by texting
So I don't come across as weak

I drink too much, it doesn't help
But numbs the pain I feel each day
And if someone asks about me
I tell them I'm ok

Each day I fight my own self worth
It exhausts me constantly
I just want to feel normal in my life
But it drains me mentally

I have cut off people in my life
Both family and friends
Thinking they don't need me
And wondering if my life should end

So, remember someone next to you
Could be struggling today
Trying to hold it all together
And fighting to be brave

My final day

It's time for me to say goodbye
To the company I've known so long
I leave the building one final time
As I'm forced now to move on

Many years we've been together
And countless laughs we've shared
The yearly Christmas parties
And the times we showed we cared

We've had our share of painful times
And lost friends along the way
But we supported one another
As we went about our day

It's hard to leave this company
It's the people I'll miss most
It's been a privilege and a pleasure
And I know that we'll stay close

I've had lots of great successes
Over many years
There's been highs and lows and challenges
As I try and hold back tears

I leave here with my head held high
And am proud of what I achieved
I did the best thing for the company
With no regrets now as I leave

So, this is now my final day
As I contemplate what's ahead
I close this door for one last time
And move on with life instead

My incredible psychologist

I'm not quite sure where to begin
I'm not sure where to start
To talk about my psychologist
When all was torn apart

I don't know where I would have been
Without her constant care
For every time I needed her
She was always there

She joined my rollercoaster ride
With compassion and concern
She gave me strength to understand
The aftermath I'd learned

She was with me at each painful step
When learning something new
Guiding me how to deal with things
And showing me what to do

She helped me navigate scenarios
That blew my mind away
She gave me tools to help support
And get me through the day

Life threw me several curveballs
They kept coming back to back
I found it hard to stay afloat
But she helped me stay on track

She's had an impact on my life
She's one I won't forget
Her support has meant the world to me
And I'm forever in her debt

My amazing support team

My colleagues, friends and family
Were amazing when news spread
They dropped everything to be with me
And supported me instead

They were there for me in so many ways
They were always by my side
So many of them came with me
On this rollercoaster ride

They called and texted me daily
They brought flowers, gifts and meals
Making sure I kept my strength up
As they all helped me heal

They listened to my story
And what I learned from day to day
When uncovering further curveballs
Reminding me to be brave

They would take away my darkness
And made me laugh until I cried
Telling jokes and funny stories
As they helped slow down this ride

They were my constant shadow
Or my shoulder to cry on
They sat with me in silence
Knowing I was not alone

They held their hands out daily
And they hugged me from afar
To lift me up and care for me
They were my shining stars

They came with me when riding
Or they took me to the beach
We would watch a morning sunrise
And realise life was still in reach

We'd take walks that went for hours
Starting at the break of day
Remembering to be grateful
And to keep my thoughts at bay

There was much more to this story
With other challenges in life
All crashing at the same time
These all kept me up at night

It was all too much to handle
These major challenges back to back
I was totally exhausted
It was hard to stay on track

But I'm so blessed and I'm so lucky
With the people close to me
I couldn't ask for better friendships
And this support is clear to see

I can't thank you all enough
For helping me through this ride
For supporting me through the hardest times
I have such love for you inside

I'm very mindful this hurt others
And this story's not all mine
We should support each other through the pain
And all heal over time

HOPE

After further research and speaking to others about their journey with depression, there is the chance of recovery. There is hope that recovery can be possible with determination, help and support.

They can come full circle and be able to live a happy and fulfilling life.

Don't ever forget – there is always hope!

Storm clouds

The sky is looking darker
As storm clouds soon appear
They're raging all around you
As you face your biggest fear

Your mind is overwhelming
With what you face each day
You can't stop these thoughts and feelings
They don't seem to go away

We know that you can fight this
And find the peace you need
If you make a plan and stick to it
For a better life to lead

There's many people to support you
A team to help you through
To listen, love and guide you
Because we care so much for you

We know there will be better days
The sky will turn to clear
Soon a bright new day will dawn
And storm clouds will disappear

There is always hope

Tell me what's happening in your life
What gets you through the day?
Are there things that trouble you?
Please tell me you're okay

Don't ever think you can't reach out
And say what's on your mind
Just talk to me, I'll listen
We'll take one day at a time

I'll take your hand and walk with you
We'll fight this dreaded fight
I'll walk this path beside you
So be strong with all your might

Don't hide behind the stigma
Please seek the help you need
It will help you fight your battle
Stand up and take the lead

It may be overwhelming
It might get really tough
I just need you to remember
You truly are enough

Life can throw some curveballs
And struggles come to hand
We'll get through these things together
Speak up and take a stand

Your friends and family need you here
You deserve the best in life
Please don't choose to end your fight
Reach out if you're in strife

I know you want the pain to stop
And sometimes you want to quit
But life won't be the same for us
Because you're part of it

We will be forever broken
We will live our lives in pain
The loss of you won't leave us
Our grief will still remain

You won't see the aftermath left behind
But I know first-hand what it's like
It's a lonely ride to hell and back
It cuts deep like a knife

There's many people who will help you
If you feel you cannot cope
Please never give up fighting
Because there is always hope

Don't be afraid to reach for help
It's the bravest thing that you can do
You're mental health's worth fighting for
And there's many people to help you

So please reach out at any time
If you feel you cannot cope
Please never give up fighting
Because there is always hope

MOVING FORWARD

Grief is not a moment in time, and it's not something you can cure. You don't move on from grief, you move forward with it.

We can be grieving, we can be happy and we can be sad all at the same time. We are continually facing countless emotions all at once—and it's exhausting! We also deal with other events in life—family or friends being ill or passing away, being unemployed or having to change jobs. Life will still continue.

We can enjoy new experiences and new relationships despite the fact we have been forced down a different path. These relationships may not have happened otherwise. We form new friendships, and we form *stronger* friendships with the ones that have supported us through the hardest times.

Sometimes, you need to take a big leap of faith and choose not to be fearful of what could go wrong but try to get enthusiastic about what could go right. This created an opportunity for me to look forward to new and exciting possibilities. Wonderful things can come your way when you least expect them to. I finally felt like I was starting to breathe again.

However, you need to remember there may be some stumbling blocks along the way. You may take one big step forward, a giant leap, but then you could take two steps back, or more and fall off the wave, just like I did.

We also need to remember how much our work affects our mental health. A bad company culture has a direct effect on the mental health of staff. We need to ensure companies create a great culture at work and ensure safe working environments. Understand the ripple effect certain behaviour has on the mental health of current staff and the ones who have left because of it.

I've taken steps forward and back in work and in life, but I still believe there are better things to come.

I remember, whatever happens in life—good or bad—life must go on!

Another rollercoaster ride

You said that you were happy
But then you texted to say
You told me it was over
And with that you walked away

You left me to pick up pieces
And deal with triggers from the past
With so many mixed emotions
I was falling down so fast

The triggers were unbearable
They brought back all my pain
I went back to the beginning
To start this ride again

I try hard to forget you
And I still see your face
You're everywhere and nowhere
But again, life's out of place

I don't know what you're looking for
You gave me a different sign
I just know that now I'm on
Another rollercoaster ride

No guarantees

I'm trying to move forward
But life still pulls me back
How can I just keep going?
How can I stay on track?

I thought life had turned a corner
I could see a brand new start
I could see new possibilities
But another breaks my heart

I now feel cold and empty
And tears have just returned
I didn't want these feelings
Another heartache now confirmed

So much of me is missing
I thought I'd come so far
But sadness seems to taunt me
And continues leaving scars

I had already been so broken
Have I not been through enough?
But another round was fired at me
I'm so tired of being tough

I'll never understand this fallout
And how the ending came to this
After many years of knowing you
It's the friendship that I'll miss

But it seems that that's all over now
I'm not sure how it can repair
I'll continue forward once again
But sadly, you're not there

Again, I'll get up fighting
With a future still to see
I'll focus on life's positives
But with no guarantees

One day at a time

I wake up to a sunrise
And contemplate the day
I think about how life is now
And all the things I want to say

I take a break and breathe again
And find peace within the past
Remembering how far I've come
And again, mend this broken heart

I have a strength from deep within
From when life's knocked me down
Once again, I get back up
And take a look around

Life will always throw a curveball
It's how you will react
It's how you will respond to it
Another lesson at my back

We all fall down from time to time
But we can get back up and fly
We need to fix our broken wings
And we can soar up to the sky

Once more I take it step by step
Like a mountain I will climb
Again, I move on with my life
And take one day at a time

When life knocks me down

Strength is letting out the tears
When there's things to cry about
But you smile and take another step
Even when there's times of doubt

Sometimes it's hard to take that leap
You need to have some faith
Because every step will help you
Make things fall into place

If you don't take that leap forward
Everything will stay the same
You need to keep progressing
And keep moving day to day

You may take a small step backwards
You may take more than one
But that is how you'll learn and grow
You'll crawl, then walk, then run

I tried to take that one step forward
Then I took several back
But I know I'm not defeated
I know I'm still on track

I'll continue moving forward
And I'll straighten out my crown
I'll have faith that things will all work out
Even when life knocks me down

The book

Life is a book we read in the present
And includes chapters from the past
But we can't keep reviewing pages
To move forward from the dark

We must turn the page of yesterday
And focus on what's in store
We have endless possibilities
A life enriched with so much more

When trying to move forward
We might get lost along the way
As we're reminded of the past again
It's not where we want to stay

Each step we take will teach us
And it's scary as we go
But think less about yesterday
And more about tomorrow

I didn't want this chapter in my life
I didn't want it in my book
As I put the past behind me
Only forward I will look

I know the future is bright for me
And I look forward to what's ahead
One day to laugh and love again
And move on with life instead

So, now I write a brand new book
With new stories made to last
The pen is in my hands now
To close this chapter of the past

You've rescued me

You came into my life
And you took me by surprise
My heart was closed and broken
But I saw something in your eyes

You gave me strength to laugh again
And a reason for my smile
You help me turn a corner
And again, life feels worthwhile

I love the way you make me feel
As my heart skips a beat
I can't explain these feelings
But I know they do run deep

I love our time together
And when you hold me tight
I know it's very early days
But somehow this just feels right

I look forward to our time ahead
And the possibilities in store
No longer looking at the past
I can't go there anymore

I'm blessed to have you in my life
And the future's bright to see
You've made me want to love again
And I feel you've rescued me

My Christmas gift to you

My gift is to bring you happiness
And put a smile upon your face
To be there for you when times get tough
Or when life gets out of place

My gift is to wipe away your pain
And kiss away your tears
It's knowing that I'm there with you
When you face your biggest fears

My gift is always listening
No matter what you need to say
Without ever passing judgement
I'll be there in every way

My gift is looking forward
As we walk this road ahead
To put the past behind us
And move on with life instead

My gift is to make sweet memories
That bring a smile across your face
To fill your heart with joy and love
That nobody can replace

My gift is giving back to you
For the constant joy you bring
And the kindness you show others
You deserve the best of things

My gift is to always make you laugh
Till tears run down our face
And knowing it's the simple things
That just can't be replaced

My gift is the things we love to do
Early morning cups of tea
And holding you upon the step
These mean so much to me

My gift is just to let you know
I love the little things you do
I love the joy you've brought to me
I'm so glad that I found you

My gift is loving you each day
As sunrise starts anew
And showing that you are my world
This is my Christmas gift to you

From the start

We knew time was getting closer
When God would call for you
It was time to stop you from your pain
He could see what you'd been through

He could see you getting tired
And that it was all too much
It was time to stop your suffering
He reached for your hand to touch

He put his arms around you
And he showed you the way
He whispered he'd take care of you
When he took you that final day

Our hearts are all so empty
As we watched you slip away
But God kept calling for you
And we couldn't make you stay

You'll never be forgotten, Mum
As you'll live inside our hearts
Thinking of sweet memories
Because we loved you from the start

Dear God

We know you have our mum now, God
You took her yesterday
We know you'll take good care of her
But there's some things we want to say

Please spend some time and talk to her
It's what she loves to do
She still loves a conversation
And she always talked of you

Please pick her flowers from time to time
She loved to smell them so
She loved the different colours
As she watched her garden grow

Please buy the paper for her
So she keeps up with the news
She loved to do the crosswords
And read other people's views

We ask that you take care of her
Be gentle 'cause she's weak
She's slower than she used to be
She's tired and she's meek

Remember that we love her, God
And we miss her so
We know you wanted her with you
But we never wanted her to go

COVID-19

A big black cloud hung over us
And was named COVID-19
We were in uncharted territory
We weren't sure what it means

This virus really changed our lives
It changed the way we lived
But once I knew it's magnitude
I could see what we'd deal with

It changed the way we went about our day
It stopped us from living life
We worked from home and had kids out of school
Many people were in strife

This virus made us fragile
We couldn't see the ones we loved
Some lost their jobs as business closed
It was so hard not to judge

We missed our friends and family
We cancelled trips and holidays
Our mental health was challenged
Affecting us in different ways

We lost loved ones to this virus
The numbers rising every day
But we had collateral damage
For the ones who lost their way

To make you stay

I sit here in the silence
I sit here all alone
I think about how life was
And remember now you're gone

Emptiness surrounds me
As I remember days with you
The fun times we spent together
And the memories that I knew

We'd been friends for many years
We travelled overseas
We laughed until the sun went down
And drank wine in the breeze

Some days are just so lonely
Remembering times with you
There's times I just can't catch my breath
Because you left too soon

I remember fun-filled moments
And when you made me smile
We had so many happy times
They made life seem worthwhile

You had hard times through COVID
And your business had to close
You seemed to lose your purpose
And this was the road you chose

I know some days you guide me through
When sadness comes my way
But our friendship was just not enough
Not enough to make you stay

Our dear friend

You fought a heavy battle
As your cancer had returned
You showed such grace and courage
As your world had been confirmed

You brought us so much sunshine
And you always had a smile
You were kind and you were caring
You made the days worthwhile

We would all catch up together
For weekends with great friends
They were full of love and laughter
And no one needed to pretend

You would stop at every doggy
And let them lick your face
It brought you so much happiness
Giving them a warm embrace

You still supported others
And helped your friends along the way
You were such a special friend to us
And we miss you every day

We still hear your laughter
It was infectious and unique
It lit up people's faces
You had that winning streak

We had our first weekend without you
But you weren't far from our minds
As we spent time reminiscing
And wishing we could turn back time

Never let her go

It was time for you to be in care
A hard decision to be made
It was the best thing for you now
As your health began to fade

We visit every single day
We don't want you to feel alone
It's not like it used to be
This room is now your home

The staff at the nursing centre
They do the best they can
And sitting in your chair each day
You said you understand

You are a favourite with the carers
You are cheeky when at play
They visit just to say, 'hello'
And it can make your day

They come and bring you ice cream
Or sing you a favourite song
They often tell you, you are handsome
And they tell you to be strong

We can see how much it means to you
We can see your eyes light up
As you banter with the carers
It seems to fill your cup

You keep looking at mum's photo
We know you miss her so
One day you'll hold her close again
And never let her go

You really are a gift

You come with me to the nursing home
Never once do you complain
And as we go each weekend
You help keep Dad entertained

You ask him lots of questions
Many queries of the past
He still has the sharpest memory
And loves the fact you asked

You get him reminiscing
And thinking how things used to be
What mischief he got up to
Or things that he's achieved

You help get him in the wheelchair
And take a spin around the grounds
Ensuring he gets sunshine
And hears the outdoor sounds

I'm so grateful that you're in my life
It's what I would have wished
I thank the one who introduced us
Because you really are a gift

Mental health in the workplace

Mental health in the workplace is so important. It can have a ripple effect on our work and other aspects of our life. In our work, it affects our productivity, the amount of time off work, staff turnover, and increased stress. In our personal lives, it affects our relationships and our physical health. So much needs to change in the workplace. Many companies don't focus on mental health appropriately. They talk the talk, but don't walk the walk. There's too much damaging conduct— toxic behaviour, blaming, yelling, bullying, gaslighting. Some people don't even seem to realise or understand what they are executing. I'm constantly told, 'You don't want to work for this company or that company.' It's a bad culture. It's a blame culture. A blame culture is a sign of weak leadership. No good can come from a blame culture; it's destructive, and it's dangerous. Yelling at staff is considered aggressive and it can be a traumatic experience for others.

Companies have staff that are unhappy, overwhelmed and exhausted. It breeds a recipe for stress and anxiety. Their hard work and long hours are rewarded with more work. So many staff have worker burnout. They can't sleep, their health is suffering, but they keep going regardless of their own health because they have commitments and families to think about. Maybe they're dealing with illness in the family, maybe they're ill themselves or they have family in care. They are working excessive hours with constant pressure and goalposts continually moving. Maybe they're juggling everything, just trying to hold it all together.

What would your staff say about your company as they leave? It's a great company, culture and experience, but time for change. Or it's toxic and unprofessional.

Leadership starts at the top. As the leader of your company, do you actually lead by example? Remember, *ALL* your staff are watching *your* behaviour. An open-door policy encourages tough conversations with management. It can help build trust and resolve issues quickly. If you do have an open-door policy, make sure you listen to your staff and take their concerns seriously. They are raising issues for a reason. It takes courage for staff to walk through your door in the first place!

How will you lead a 'positive and inspiring only' environment so employees can feel they are doing a good job and can care for their families the way they want to? If your family member lived with a mental illness, wouldn't you want someone protecting them? I know I would. Why should anyone have to work in a toxic environment? Employees don't sign up for that!

What will you change to ensure your company is a successful, happy and safe environment for everyone?

Your leadership style is what *you* will be remembered for. What kind of legacy do you want to leave behind?

The workplace

The workplace can be so stressful
When deadlines and goals come first
We can easily forget our mental health
When we're so focused on our work

There is a constant pressure
And many last-minute requests
With limited time to actually finish them
Work can cause us so much stress

The goal posts will keep on moving
When another request comes down the line
When you will have to change direction
And again with limited time

But it's important to remember
That our mental health's at risk
When we're not taking care of it
We simply can't perform our best

Companies should create a safe environment
That openly talks on mental health
Offering their staff resources
To ensure they have some help

Talk to someone if you're struggling
Ask your doctor for advice
Use the tools the company offers you
So your mental health doesn't pay the price

We're all guilty of putting the workplace first
And not what's most important in our lives
But when life's cut short, what's the point?
Because all we've lost, is time

We're not family

Many companies say, 'We're family'
But that's not exactly true
Companies may want a family culture
But our family isn't you

You might want a family dynamic
Of support and trust and care
A healthy relationship with colleagues
But our family isn't there

We go home to our family
They're not the ones keeping us at work
Pressuring us to put up with behaviours
Or killing our self-worth

When companies say, 'We're family'
We feel pressure to accept
Mistreatment and poor boundaries
And putting our health at neglect

A family doesn't 'let you go'
When the times are tough
They help support and guide you
And they remind you 'you're enough'

So we might work together
Spending many hours naturally
We're colleagues, workmates and even friends
But, we're not family

A good company culture

A good company culture should feel like a warm embrace
Staff should feel safe and secure
They should have support when in the workplace
Or with personal issues to endure

A good company culture is collaborative
Showing the way when you are lost
Helping you reach your full potential
And not doing business at any cost

A good company culture is supportive
Making you feel like you belong
It gives you hope when you're feeling down
And helps you to be strong

A good company culture is inclusive
And welcomes new employees
Regardless of their backgrounds
They should put everyone at ease

A good company culture is fair and equitable
Staff are rewarded for their work
They set clear expectations
And ensure staff aren't overworked

A good company culture is conversations
Giving staff the chance to learn and grow
They are challenged to be the best they can
And to reach their full potential

A good company culture is transparent
With management communications to the staff
On key decisions and the future
Not giving information by the half

A good company culture works together
And is productive as a team
Ensuring staff are motivated
With a happy and healthy theme

A good company culture is rewarding
Where staff can see the work they do
It is really making a difference
And the company actually follows through

A good company culture has fun and laughter
And everyone understands their roles
As the team works towards a purpose
And achieving company goals

Can you see the forest for the trees?

What does your company culture look like?
Have you found that common ground?
Is your team excited to come to work
When Monday morning comes around?

Companies have a responsibility
To provide a safe and healthy space
Please leave the egos at the door
And create a happy place

Does your team see you as a leader
Inspiring them to be their best
Giving a vision for the future
And recognising team success?

Do you set clear expectations
Or do the goal posts always move?
Do staff find it hard to please you
Because you always disapprove?

Are you too engrossed in other details?
Are you focusing on one thing?
Do you constantly blame each other?
What value do you bring?

Do you just focus on the top line
Or do you understand the weeds?
If you don't care about the issues
You're not likely to succeed

Have you caused some of these issues
Because you didn't listen to your team
And went against their judgement
Now the issues are extreme?

How do you help support your staff
When they raise up their hands?
Do you actually hear what they are saying
Or do you just make more demands?

How have you contributed
When promoting staff within?
Do you help to guide and mentor them
Or just let them sink or swim?

Do you go and see your customers
And get insights first-hand?
To see what sales are up against
And really try to understand?

Do you trust your staff to do the job
You hired them to do?
Do you know when to apologise
Or give credit when it's due?

Do you have their backs when times are tough
Or do you throw them to the wolves?
Do you find a way to let others shine
Or just think about yourselves?

Do you truly know your leadership team
And how they treat the staff?
How they treat you and other leaders
Might be a very different path

Do you actually support mental health
Or just pretend you do?
Are you just ticking all the boxes
Or do you actually follow through?

Do you know if staff are suffering
With stress and anxiety
With constant worker burnout
Or inequality?

Do you have enough staff in each department
Or are you far too lean
Putting all that extra pressure
And extra hours on your team?

How much money has been wasted
Due to constant staffing needs?
The loss of knowledge and experience
And of company expertise?

Do you know what people talk about
Or the word upon the street?
What would they say about your company?
Would they want to join your team?

Do you realise not every manager
Should be responsible for a team?
They should not be managing people
Or there may be a toxic theme

Your staff are your biggest assets
Without them where would you be?
Success will always follow
With happy and valued employees

Can you really see the issues
In the team you thought you knew?
Can you see some of these issues
Might actually, be you?

This one might be hard to answer
But it does need to be said
Are you the right person in the driver's seat
Or should you step aside instead?

Can you read yourself within this forest
Or will you just focus on the trees?
Do you have the self-awareness
To make the changes that you need?

It's all part of health and safety
And understanding all the risks
Promoting health and wellness
And ensure no bullying exists

Someone's life might be in crisis
They could be treading on thin ice
You could be triggering past emotions
And causing many sleepless nights

So, to all the 'leaders' out there
Please take a step back and see
What does your culture REALLY look like?
Can you see the forest for the trees?

No more sleepless nights

It was many years of being tired
From all the sleepless nights
As my brain was overloaded
From these curveballs in my life

It was the constant morning wake ups
With my frequent racing thoughts
Initially with such trauma
And the pain that this had brought

But then it became my workload
And the constant pressure day to day
Meeting unrealistic expectations
That never seemed to go away

This was not what I signed up for
Losing so much personal time
Working late each night and weekends
It was such a long, hard climb

I worked so hard both day and night
But never felt it was enough
I never felt respected
Turning up to work was tough

I chose to leave this company
With my eyes set on new sights
I have so much stress released now
And there's no more sleepless nights

Friends for life

It's not the same without my team mates
And I've felt lost along the way
But even though I chose to leave
I miss them everyday

We've created such strong friendships
And we know each other's pain
We've always helped each other
And supported through the strain

We adjusted through the workload
When there was no end in site
Talking on the phone together
While working late into the night

This helped keep us going
And we could laugh along the way
It always kept our spirits up
As we went on day to day

This team is all so caring
They're passionate and kind
They work hard every single day
And they are the best you'll find

We are all like sisters now
And we share a special bond
We'll stay close in each other's lives
For tomorrow and beyond

I'm so blessed I met these team mates
And they came into my life
It's something that I'm grateful for
Because we're now friends for life

Keep on searching

I have a wonderful man in my life
Amazing family and friends
And many things to be grateful for
But some days, seem impossible
There's been so much heartache
So many things in life have changed
Things I've had no control over
I now live with anxiety, which has been fuelled
through different scenarios over recent years
I've dealt with things I shouldn't have had to deal with
I've had to make decisions I shouldn't have had to make
I've been collateral damage when I didn't deserve to be
I feel I have no purpose
I don't know where I belong
Right now, I'm lost
I'm looking for something I cannot seem to find
But I'll keep on searching

Rainbows and unicorns

If only life could be like a child's mind
Expressive, innocent and free
Filled with fairy dust and moonbeams
And all those fun things life should be

If we could always see full colour
Instead of black and white
If we supported one another more
Instead of picking fights

If we could work together
And hear each other's point of view
If we just listened to each other
We may learn something new

If we could show each other kindness
And give each other hope
We don't know each other's story
They could be on a slippery slope

If we could understand each other's troubles
And feel each other's pain
We come together through the hard times
And see the scars that will remain

Curveballs affect us all in different ways
It's this story that's called life
Let's wrap our arms around each other
Instead of causing strife

We all have the right to tell our story
Sharing what or how we feel
Understanding all the chapters
And come together as we heal

Let's just support each other
And make sure everyone belongs
If only life could really be
All rainbows and unicorns

95 not out!

Today it is your birthday, Dad
You turn 95 years young
Born in 1928
Was when it all begun

You met our mum at a tennis match
And married in 1955
With her raised seven children
Managing to keep us all alive

Nine people lived in one small house
But somehow, we made it work
There was some constant chaos
And some days we went berserk

We didn't grow up very wealthy
But we went to private schools
You and Mum made sacrifices
And we were breaking rules

You watched us all grow into adults
With many things that we've achieved
We know you're proud of all of us
And the adults we grew to be

You have eight amazing grandchildren
Four great-grandchildren now in place
They're the ones who bring you joy
And put a smile upon your face

You shouldn't really have a favourite
But we quietly know you do
She's the one who makes you cry
When she comes to visit you

You enjoy sports like the cricket
You know what it's all about
Celebrate your birthday innings, Dad
Because you're 95 not out!

The sunrise

The sun rises over the ocean
A palette of golden tones
Of reds and yellows and oranges
As I take it in alone

What a beautiful sight to start the day
It's so peaceful and so quiet
With the sky in all its glory
In the calming morning light

The waves are slowly rolling in
And breaking on the shore
At this time of the morning
I couldn't ask for more

The sun has finished rising
As blue sky scatters all around
With clouds that look like cotton wool
I enjoy the calm surrounds

I love to watch the sunrise
And the seagulls now at play
It reminds me of the simple things
And a perfect way to start the day

Just smile

Smiling is like a superpower
It can help anxiety
It can help increase endorphins
And release stress naturally

A smile can lift our moods up
And cause a positive ripple effect
Which makes us all feel happy
And helps people connect

So, when you see someone in passing
Even someone you don't know
Show a little act of kindness
And just smile and say, 'hello'

The simple things in life

Watching a morning sunrise
Before you start your day
The smell of coffee brewing
To get you on your way

Dancing through the ocean waves
And running through the sand
Feeling it between our toes
While walking hand in hand

The sound of waves at night time
As they crash onto the beach
Is so very therapeutic
As you dream and fall asleep

Sitting around a fire pit
And watching embers glow
Having fresh clean sheets to sleep in
With your favourite pillow

Watching stars by moonlight
When night time comes around
In the silence of the darkness
When no one makes a sound

Listening to those special songs
That take you back in time
Bringing back the memories
Reminding you of other times

The welcome from your dog each time
You open up the door
Especially after a long hard day
They couldn't love you any more

The smell of fresh cut grass on a summer's day
Or making someone smile
These are all some little things
That can make our day worthwhile

So, pick your favourite things to do
And follow this advice
Either by yourself or with some friends
Enjoy the simple things in life

Life is a gift

Life is precious and it's a gift
But in a heartbeat it can change
It's something we should cherish
As we go about our day

We should make time for what's important
And for the ones who mean the most
Never taking time for granted
As we hold our loved ones close

Every moment is a blessing
Each breath we take, a miracle
Some lose this gift too soon in life
Which can be unbearable

We should remember we are fortunate
As we take a breath each day
Be grateful for this precious gift
For good things to come your way

Let's make the most of living
And ensure we have a blast
Keep reaching for the stars each day
And live each day like it's our last

Yesterday

Yesterday is a day gone by
It's time to let it go
To focus on the present
And think about tomorrow

Yesterday may have had some challenges
It may have had regrets
But today it is a brand new day
And it's time to start afresh

Yesterday may have had some memories
That may be good and bad
But today has new potential
With a new day to make a stand

So, just let go of yesterday
And move forward from the past
Embrace each new day calling
As time moves by so fast

Yesterday has passed and today is now
Tomorrow is a mystery
So make the most of every minute
Because soon it's history

You need to live in every moment
And just enjoy the ride
Don't dwell on things you can't control
As time's not always on your side

Make the most of what you have right now
And be grateful for each day
Stop wishing you could change the past
Because you can't change yesterday

I believe

I believe life can be difficult
I believe it can be cruel
I believe in possibilities
And breaking all the rules

I believe that strength will see me through
When life gets pretty tough
I believe that I am worthy
And I believe I am enough

I believe in kissing slowly
And holding loved ones close
I believe in talking openly
About what means the most

I believe in love and laughter
I believe in destiny
I believe there's brighter days ahead
And there's better things for me

I believe in loving with all my heart
The one who means the most
And holding onto one another
When each day comes to a close

I believe in saying sorry
When you know you have done wrong
I believe music changes everything
When you hear your favourite song

I believe we all can make mistakes
And we make people upset
We should fix things while we have the chance
So, we don't live with regret

I believe people make bad choices
But it's not really who they are
It only makes them human
They shouldn't be forever scarred

I believe in second chances
If you've learned from your mistakes
To prove things will be different
And believe a heart won't break

I believe that life is just too short
You should tell people where they stand
About how much they mean to you
In case you never get the chance

I believe in watching sunrises
As we start a brand new day
I believe in being grateful
When good things come our way

I believe in watching stars at night
When it's peaceful and it's quiet
We calm our mind and reminisce
About the good things in our life

I believe in showing kindness
And treating others with respect
We don't know what they've been through
So just be compassionate

I believe good friends are hard to find
And we may have just a few
To love, support and make us smile
As they go through life with you

I believe in having friends around
Who make you laugh until you cry
I believe in making miracles
And reaching for the sky

I believe one day stars will align
And all things will fall in place
So that life will be amazing
With so many dreams to chase

How you can help support someone living with depression

- Firstly, acknowledge that depression is a condition, they are not just 'being sad'.
- Educate yourself about depression and understand how the easiest of tasks can be completely overwhelming.
- Remember, depression is often invisible.
- Be a good listener and really hear what they are saying. Please let them do the talking. It's not about you!
- Never say, 'I know how you feel' if you don't live with depression. Again, it's not about you and no one can ever know exactly how someone else feels! That can come across as condescending.
- Never say things like, 'Stop being sad', or 'Get over it', or 'I get sad too'. It's not even close to the same thing or realistically possible.
- Have patience and understanding and try to empathise as best you can.
- Depression is a rollercoaster—there will be good days and bad. Stay with them.
- Constantly validate them and build them up. Remind them they are loved, wanted, needed, a good person, etc.
- If they start to withdraw, find a way to spend time with them. Don't just shut them out.
- Ask how you can help them and what they need from you.

- Don't correct or contradict them. While their depression may colour their thinking, don't behave as if you know them better than they know themselves.
- Sufferers are not lazy, but depression can paralyse them.
- Help them to understand the importance of professional help and support them through it. They may need guidance to get started.
- If you are supporting someone living with depression, put all emergency numbers in your telephone.
- Be mindful that supporting a loved one with depression can be very challenging and draining. It's okay to feel helpless or powerless. Lay people are not equipped to take this on alone and do the work of a professional, so if you are supporting someone, please also seek support systems to assist you.

Useful resources

www.lifeline.org.au
www.beyondblue.org.au
www.blackdoginstitute.org.au
www.gotcha4life.org
www.headspace.org.au
www.mensline.org.au
www.ruok.org.au
www.lifeline.org.nz
www.whatsup.co.nz
www.outline.org.nz
www.youthline.co.nz

Please also search for resources within your own country.

Helplines

Australia:
Lifeline 13 11 14 or text 0477 13 11 14
Suicide Call Back Service 1300 659 467
Beyond Blue 1300 224 636
Headspace 1800 650 890 for
young people 12-25 years
Kids Help Line 1800 55 1800
Men's Helpline Australia 1300 78 99 78
Open Arms – Veterans & Families
Counselling 1800 011 046

New Zealand:

Lifeline 0800 543 354 or
free text 4357 (HELP)
Suicide Crisis Helpline 0508 828 865
Depression Helpline 0800 111 757
or free text 4202
Kidsline 0800 543 754 for
children up to 18 years
Samaritans Aotearoa 0800 726 666
What's Up 0800 942 878 for
children 5-18 years
Youthline 0800 376 633 or free text 234

In any country:

- Ask for help, talk to family and friends.
- Talk to your doctor and ask to be referred to a counsellor, psychologist or psychiatrist, depending on your needs.
- Visit your local hospital.
- Find out help options and resources in your local area.

About the author

Jo Woodhouse lives in Sydney, Australia.

She has mainly worked in the healthcare industry, but now that she has found the love of writing, she has drafted two children's books, which she also hopes to publish.

When she's not working, you will find her spending time with family and friends, with a paintbrush in hand, on long distance walks, or lazing on the beach in summer.

*'We should not forget that we
are all human and fall
from time to time.*

*It is easy to fall and hard to get back up,
but that is where resilience is forged,
and growth occurs.'*

Sibel Terhaar

www.ingramcontent.com/pod-product-compliance
Lightning Source LLC
Chambersburg PA
CBHW051438270326
41931CB00019B/3469